The Journey

The Journey

A Family's Firsthand ALS Account

MITCHELL BRENT SPIEGEL

ISBN: 1514654113
ISBN 13: 9781514654118
Library of Congress Control Number: 2015911249
CreateSpace Independent Publishing Platform
North Charleston, South Carolina

Acknowledgment

This book is dedicated to my mom, Judy Blair Spiegel, who passed away from amyotrophic lateral sclerosis (ALS) in September 2014. My mom was a truly amazing woman whose strength, bravery, and resolve were an inspiration to all who knew her. Her beauty, elegance, warmth, and grace touched those who had the privilege of being part of her life. Without question, my life and our family's lives will never be the same without her—she was a force of nature. My mother and I shared a lot of life's experiences over the years, and I learned many lessons from her.

My mom helped instill in me the discipline and confidence to succeed and compete. She gave me the wisdom to learn from failure; she highlighted the importance of hard work and a strong ethic; she stressed to me that I should say what I mean and mean what I say; and, most importantly, she instilled in me the importance of family, sacrifice, respect, privacy, and loyalty. I will be forever grateful to her for the relationship that we shared and the life's lessons that she taught me.

I would like to thank my wife for her support, empathy, love, and patience and my children for being a source of inspiration and strength. Finally, I would like to thank Dr. Georgia Witkin, for the encouragement and guidance to complete this project.

Foreword

ALS, or, as it's better known, Lou Gehrig's disease, is a disease that has recently received a lot of national attention, thanks to the Ice Bucket Challenge. Prior to my mom's diagnosis and the Ice Bucket Challenge, the book *Tuesdays with Morrie* was my primary source of ALS information. I do not work in the medical field, so this disease was a bit of a mystery to me—I knew a little bit about Lou Gehrig and his issues, but not very much. Suffice it to say that I now know much more about the disease and the devastation that it causes.

Type *ALS* into Google, and it does not take long to figure out that it is a disease that affects the nerve cells in the brain and spinal cord that control voluntary muscle movement (like talking, swallowing, walking, breathing, etc.). ALS is a formidable disease, one in which a patient's functioning mind is eventually entombed in his or her own paralyzed body.

According to the ALS Association, ALS most commonly strikes people between the ages of forty and seventy. It is estimated that there are as many as thirty thousand people in the United States who have the disease at any given time. ALS does not discriminate by gender, race, geography, ethnicity, or socioeconomic status—it is an equal opportunity menace. The ALS Association reports as follows:

- "Each year roughly fifty-six hundred people in the United States are diagnosed with ALS.

- The average life expectancy of an ALS patient is between two and five years from the time of diagnosis.
- More than half of all ALS patients live more than three years after diagnosis.
- About 20 percent of ALS patients live five years or more, up to 10 percent will survive more than ten years, and about 5 percent will survive twenty years after diagnosis."[1]

I started sketching the outline for this book shortly after my family met with the hospice provider at my mom's apartment. At first, the book started out as a way to distract myself from my mom's failing health. After my mom passed away, this book became a form of therapy for me—a way that I could express the intensity of the emotional roller coaster that I had been strapped into since June 11, 2013 (the date my mom was diagnosed with ALS). It was a medium where I could vent my frustration and express my pain. I wrote in the early mornings, late at night, and with whatever free time I could steal on the weekends when I was not spending time with my wife and three children. Midway through the writing process, I realized that perhaps this book could help others manage and prepare for this unfortunate journey. The more people I told about my book idea, the more I realized that I should continue to write and complete this book.

The purpose of this book is to help others going through the ALS journey. Unfortunately, when my family went through this process, we did not have a resource like this to help prepare us. This book is just that, a layman's (non-medical) firsthand account of how ALS impacts a patient and his or her family and a guide to steps that can be taken to mitigate some of the foreseeable challenges that we encountered. No punches are pulled—I do not "toe the party line" about the disease, doctors, clinics, and health-care system. I try not to sugarcoat the relevant information, my frustrations during the process, or how the story ends; my goal was to be as direct as possible. Looking back, I wish I had found a resource like this—my family may have been better prepared for what was on the horizon, and maybe we could have avoided some of the "fire drills" my family endured.

At the end of the day, it is unlikely that the outcome would have materially changed for my mother. However, we could have been better prepared to deal with the challenges presented as the disease progressed and my mother's health descended. During this time, I found solace reading *Tuesdays with Morrie*. I read the book several years ago and reread it shortly after my mom was diagnosed. I thought that I had a sense of what was coming down the pike, but the truth is that unless you have experienced ALS firsthand, it's hard to appreciate what this disease does. Mention ALS to a physician and his or her response and expression says it all. Usually, the doctor's face drops, and an expression of pity and sympathy takes over. I recently had an annual checkup with my dermatologist. When I told him about my mother, he said, "I think ALS is the worst of the worst of diseases."

If you don't know already, there is no cure for ALS, and no one survives ALS. There is barely a medical protocol to delay the disease's progression. It is more like an observation protocol where a patient's descent is documented and observed as the signals from the brain stop reaching a patient's muscles and extremities.

Imagine watching a car crash in slow motion. You know the ultimate outcome and are powerless to change the events. At the end of the day, all patients die from the disease. Each patient's story is different—some have a more typical manifestation of the disease in their extremities, while others experience the effects of ALS in their swallowing and breathing regions, controlled by the bulbar area of the brain. The progression varies with each patient. Factors like age, race, and where they live all lead to unique, highly differentiated experiences.

My mother had progressive bulbar palsy (PBP). Some neurologists consider PBP to be a subset of ALS, which will eventually develop into full-blown ALS. In my mind, it's truly a distinction without difference. ALS or PBP—either one sucks, and both end the same way: the patient dies.

For those of you that did not know my mom, she was a beautiful, elegant woman. After she passed away, many people commented, "She was a lady." Her beauty was both inside and out. She was generous, warm, passionate, and someone that people genuinely liked being around. She was a devoted wife to my father, an amazing sister, an exemplary aunt, an exciting companion, a courageous patient, a great cook and entertainer, a loyal, reliable friend to many, a dependable mother-in-law, the best "Mima" in the world to her six grandkids, and an extraordinary mother. She set the bar very high in each and every role that she filled. As I learned through this journey, ALS may take a life, but it does not necessarily end a relationship.

Author's Note

Throughout this book, I have changed all of the doctors' names. "Dr. X----", "Dr. Y----" as well as the "phantom pulmonologist" are all doctors that my family encountered during our journey.

Table of Contents

One

The ALS Diagnosis

At this time, there is no specific bright-line medical test for ALS—there are no confirmatory biopsies, X-rays, or blood tests available. The ALS diagnosis comes after the doctor has pretty much eliminated all other potential diagnoses.

My mom was officially diagnosed with ALS on June 11, 2013. After enduring roughly eighteen months of increased fatigue, loss of appetite, weight loss, some slurred speech, and breathing challenges, she finally heard a neurologist make the diagnosis. During the eighteen months before the official diagnosis, my mom had every possible test out there: CAT scans, MRI scans, blood panels upon blood panels, and X-rays. She visited doctors from all disciplines: gastroenterologists (GI); ear, nose, and throat (ENT) specialists; pulmonary specialists; and others. Because there is no specific bright-line test for ALS, the diagnosis comes after the doctor has eliminated all other potential diseases.

Prior to my mom's diagnosis, in December of 2012, some doctors suggested that my mom had a severe case of silent acid reflux. The doctor prescribed medication and instructed my mom to stay upright for two hours after eating each meal. Yet her appetite continued to decline, she lost weight, her speech became increasingly slurred, and her energy level descended. She also started to cough and had several choking episodes on her own saliva and while eating. Up until June 11, 2013, supposedly no doctor knew what was wrong.

Finally, in the spring of 2013, my mom was referred to Dr. X---- a neurologist from the Cornell Medical Center. I remember thinking how odd it was to be referred to a neurologist—did my mom have a brain tumor? I went online and saw the types of diseases that neurologists diagnose: ALS, Alzheimer's, and Parkinson's—quite the rogue's gallery. I had no idea what a motor neuron disease was, but I learned fast. Nothing made sense until June 2013. I vividly recall Dr. X---- giving my mom the ALS diagnosis. "I'm so sorry to say that you have ALS." Shock, confusion, sadness, and despair engulfed us. My mom said that she was going to die. After a short period of awkward silence, I responded that we all are going to die someday, and this diagnosis did not mean that life ended or that tomorrow one of us would not be killed by a bus, a cab jumping the curb, or an accident at a construction site. In retrospect, my mom had just received her death sentence. The only question was when the executioner would set her date—there would not be any stay granted.

After hearing such a dreadful diagnosis, the initial response was that there was some type of mistake. So we obtained a second opinion and even a third opinion. One of our extended family members was a doctor at the Mayo Clinic; we sent all of my mom's test results to him for his review and for him to share with his colleagues in the neurology department. They felt that the EMG tests and physical symptoms were indeed consistent with ALS. My aunt's husband, Dr. Robert Rose (Dr. Robert), a cardiologist/internist, also reviewed the results.

We then visited the ALS clinic at Columbia University. An EMG test administered by our neurologist was both painful and uncomfortable, so much so that when our family went for a second opinion, my mom declared that she would not take those tests again and that the ALS clinic would need to rely on the first set of tests to confirm the diagnosis. We met the ALS specialist who published "the ALS book" for our consultation (and I believe that was the last time he was involved with my mother's care). "The ALS book," titled *Amyotrophic Lateral Sclerosis: A Guide for Patients and Families,* is a comprehensive 475-page book about the diagnosis, treatment, and progression of the disease. I found the book to be overwhelming and likely better suited for a medical person than a nonmedical person. My mother's diagnosis was a slight variant of ALS. The doctor said that my mom had progressive bulbar palsy (PBP)—essentially a subset of ALS. After scanning the web and learning about PBP, it was clear to me that this was a distinction without difference—sort of like looking at a color and debating whether the shade is navy blue or midnight blue.

I learned that ALS is a hypermetabolic disease, which means that the body burns, or metabolizes, calories at a faster rate than those without ALS. So if a woman typically consumes 1,500 calories to maintain her weight, a woman diagnosed with ALS would need to consume 2,250 calories to maintain her weight. The body is basically burning calories at one and a half times the normal rate. The loss of muscle mass and weight can accelerate the condition, forcing each nerve cell to work more muscles than before. The ALS patient needs to keep up the caloric intake to prevent the body from burning up the muscles to get calories.

For my family, helping my mother was made more challenging because my mom was a private person. She did not want to disclose her condition outside of her family and a few very close friends. Obviously, each patient deals with the diagnosis differently. My mom did not want a pity party. She wanted to manage the condition on her own terms. We respected her decision. Accordingly, we did not disclose my mom's ALS diagnosis. We told people that my mom had a ministroke, which caused her speech issues and weight loss.

Looking back, this is one of the few decisions that I wish we had handled differently. I compare my mom's decision to keep her diagnosis private to a choice made by a colleague to share that his spouse had stage-four cervical cancer. Instead of concocting a story about his wife's health, he inquired via a broadly distributed e-mail whether anyone knew of someone who had gone through a similar experience. In my opinion, sharing a common experience could be helpful and lead to informative discussions. As it turned out, my colleague met someone whose wife had been recently diagnosed with a similar cervical condition. The two husbands were able to learn from each other about what was on the horizon, as one wife had the surgery first and the other wife had the chemotherapy regiment first.

My mom's nonmedical team was deep, strong, and supportive. It had to be because ALS drains the emotional, physical, and financial resources of the primary caregivers. Much of the frontline duties were managed by Roy, my mom's boyfriend of eight years (who opted into this journey after we learned of ALS's destructive path). In addition to Roy, me, and my brother Greg, my mom's team consisted of her daughters-in-law, her sister Cyndee, and Dr. Robert along with her broad circle of friends—some lifelong that knew the diagnosis, and some who did not and did not seem to care what her condition was but wanted to support my mom and be her friend regardless of her underlying condition.

Two

The Early Days

My mom was a social person and well liked by her peers. As mentioned earlier, she was also a very private person. As a friend, my mom was compassionate, trustworthy, loyal, and discreet. She was an excellent sounding board and dispensed solid advice. These qualities drew people to her and led to so many lifelong friendships. I believe it was the reason so many of her friends continued to support her unconditionally (even without full disclosure regarding her illness).

While my mom decided not to go public with her illness, her friends knew that something was amiss, especially after her voice failed to return after the "ministroke." I was particularly touched by her group of card-playing friends that would come to the house on the weekends and play bridge and canasta with my mom. These card games were six to eight-hour marathons and amazingly, despite my mom eventually losing her ability to speak, the card games continued.

Communication takes many forms, and since my mom's mental faculties continued to be razor sharp, she could still write down her card moves. In solidarity with my mom, the card ladies spoke less, shared pictures, and wrote down card moves. They played cards, had lunch, and celebrated their children's and grandchildren's accomplishments. On more than one occasion, they even allowed my daughter to sit in on some card hands as she sat on my mother's lap.

I'm not sure whether it was my mom's desire for privacy that stirred inquiry and interest in her condition or the morbid curiosity that some of her contemporaries must have been experiencing as they considered their own mortality, but some of the rumor mongering during my mom's illness led to some curious and awkward conversations.

I remember being accosted at my seven-year-old son's baseball game by my mom's contemporary. I was coaching third base, and this woman started peppering me with questions. I wondered how this woman could actually think that she had the standing (My mom and she were not that close.) to ask these questions and that I would actually answer. Needless to say, I did not discuss my mom's condition with this woman. Yet, after this brief exchange on the baseball diamond, she told her friends that I confirmed my mom's diagnosis, a blatant lie that forced me to recount my conversation, or lack thereof, to my mom.

Not surprisingly, about seventeen months later, at a restaurant, this same woman started bombarding my wife and me at dinner with questions about my mom. This woman was sharing a dinner with her husband and grandchild. Having learned from my first interaction with her, and after evading multiple inquires and ducking and weaving her questions for what seemed like an hour, I finally turned to her and said, "I hope that you enjoy your dinner with your husband and grandchild," and turned away. People are interesting creatures. While I don't believe she had malice in her heart, her sense of boundaries really seemed out of whack.

Three

The Course of Treatment or Lack Thereof...

From my vantage point, the medical profession knows very little about ALS. Accordingly, the medical game plan to combat the disease is virtually nonexistent. What does exist is a maintenance and observation protocol. Outside of the one approved medication, Rilutek, which is supposed to extend an ALS patient's life for several months, the primary elements of care consist of focusing on a patient's caloric intake and utilizing various breathing aids.

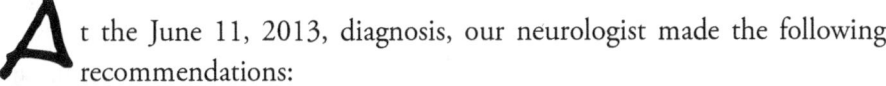

At the June 11, 2013, diagnosis, our neurologist made the following recommendations:

- Put in the percutaneous endoscopic gastrostomy feeding tube (PEG) to ensure a pathway to consume calories and reduce choking risk going forward.
- Prescribed Rilutek—the only FDA-approved drug for ALS. Our neurologist informed us that some medical studies suggest that Rilutek

can extend an ALS patient's life by several months.[2] (But it is worth considering the quality of the life extended over this period.)

- Talked about prescribing a medicine (Mestanon) to help improve the communication between the nerves and the muscles; however, Mestanon increases saliva production, which increases the choking risk.
- Encouraged my mom to take another breathing test with her pulmonologist to set a baseline of her breathing function.

The plan was to return in a week after completing the breathing test, and he recommended monthly appointments moving forward. Our family met with the neurologist on June 19, 2013, for the follow-up meeting. The following recommendations were made:

- Put in the PEG to ensure a pathway to consume calories and reduce choking risk. The doctor recommended two doctors to perform the surgical procedure.
- Get a second opinion.
- Continue the use of antidepressant medication.
- Remember that calories were key and that concerns about elevated cholesterol levels were truly secondary in nature. The translation was that my mom could eat whatever she wanted; the fattier and heavier the better. Milk shakes, ice cream, fried foods—you name it, all were approved and encouraged.

After reviewing the results of my mom's June breathing test, the neurologist noted a decline in my mom's breathing function compared to the February 2013 breathing test. He suggested using a device commonly used for sleep apnea, a BiPap machine, to ensure that her lungs got worked out and continued the process of taking fresh oxygen in and pushing carbon dioxide out.

We discussed the different care options. The neurologist supported getting a second diagnosis and recommended the ALS clinic at Columbia University. He compared and contrasted the pros and cons of a clinic setting versus staying with a single practitioner who would quarterback and organize all of the related medical services. Moreover, he was not aware of any clinical trials going on that could potentially help my mom's condition.

As our journey progressed, we did hear of several clinical trials (one in Boston at Mass General and one in Michigan at the University of Michigan) that were testing stem cells to combat the more traditional form of ALS (non-bulbar) in the spinal cord. Unfortunately, no clinical trials were available to address the bulbar version of the disease. The doctor's recommendation was to choose *either* a clinical care setting or a single practitioner setting, but not both, to avoid having too many cooks in the kitchen. He felt sharing medical records and recommendations could prove to be difficult, and there would be inefficiencies in accessing medical systems and records.

My mom took it all in and then decided, however, to pursue both avenues, so we visited the ALS clinic at Columbia on a quarterly basis and maintained our monthly appointments with our diagnosing neurologist. I personally found the clinic setting experience underwhelming at best. At each session, she would meet with a speech therapist, a respiratory therapist, a physical therapist, a social worker, and the attending physician (not the doctor that wrote the "ALS book" and made the original PBP diagnosis. In fact, over the next fifteen months, we never saw him again). Representatives of each medical discipline would come into the examining room, meet with my mom, basically extract the relevant information that they were tracking among their patients, and then leave, and we would repeat the same ritual every three months. In between, we could e-mail questions to the clinic if needed. Each clinical session took between two and three hours.

The setting was impersonal. The clinic did not provide the same level of medical access and comfort as visiting a physician once a month. Moreover, when I had a question related to my mom's medication, I had to e-mail the question to the social worker at the ALS clinic. The social worker then forwarded my medical question to the doctor, who eventually responded (several days later) via a secure e-mail—not a phone call. This was a very disappointing impersonal exchange. It made me feel like the doctors considered my mom to be just another number in the clinic. I think it is reasonable to expect human interaction when following up with a doctor. I compare this experience to my experience when I had to call Dr. X----. Each time, Dr. X---- returned my call in a timely manner and spoke with me on the phone.

In the clinical setting, there was no one quarterbacking my mom's care. I felt as if we were on a rudderless ship floating in the morass of this disease that would get boarded and inspected and then left out in the ocean after our quarterly exam was completed. It would have been helpful to have a point person, someone clearly in charge, who would have overseen my mom's dietary intake and respiratory progress in real time. That's why I found having a monthly medical appointment to be important—it provided steady, consistent, and responsive medical access.

However, even in the monthly setting, no one was really playing quarterback either. I expected a detailed summary of her weight trend, some muscle strength analysis, etc., but there was none of that. There were some physical strength exercises and tests that the doctor performed at each meeting, and that was about it. Since caloric intake and respiratory performance are so essential to managing the disease, someone has to be the point person and manager of this critical information.

One of the most frustrating aspects about this process was the lack of directness and clarity at each medical meeting—whether in the clinical or monthly setting. My brother and I tried to frame my mom's health in terms of a baseball game by asking each doctor to what inning (out of nine innings) they thought the disease had progressed. Most responses were a version of "it's very hard to say because the disease impacts each patient differently." Maybe the doctors did not want to destroy the hope we had or take away the sliver of optimism we had held onto since the beginning of this journey.

So let me lay out two key takeaways if you are dealing with ALS. Both are critical, and I wish we had heard these salient points each time we visited the ALS clinic or had our monthly ALS doctor appointment. One is regarding nutrition and the other is regarding the BiPap machine:

1. Take in as many calories as possible, and if that means embracing the PEG sooner rather than later, then so be it. If that means eating foods

that you don't like or don't taste great but are rich in calories, just do it! Take the time to figure out what PEG delivery method (discussed in chapter 4) works best for the individual patient. It will be a frustrating process with a lot of trial and error. Over time, the PEG feeding will be the patient's sole nutritional source. Losing weight accelerates a patient's medical descent as the body eventually starts to burn up muscle to feed itself, and the cycle of fatigue gets worse and worse.

2. Plain and simple, carbon dioxide retention can kill a patient. The BiPap machine is critical, because it takes the carbon dioxide out of the patient's body. We were told that the BiPap machine would help with my mom's declining energy and labored breathing—both of which were true, but the BiPap machine also reduces carbon dioxide building up in a patient's bloodstream. The BiPap fits on a patient's face like a fighter pilot's mask, and it helps patients breathe and continue to exercise their breathing muscles. Air flows through the mask and helps expand the depth of the patient's breath (bringing oxygen into the lungs) and then helps the patient to exhale (releasing the carbon dioxide). As the PEG becomes the patient's sole source of nutrition, over time, the BiPap will become the patient's sole source of noninvasive ventilation (before the tracheostomy tube procedure – "trache").

Four

The Percutaneous Endoscopic Gastrostomy Tube (PEG) and Why It's So Important

Initially, the PEG is meant to supplement typical mouth feedings, but over time, as the swallowing/bulbar muscles weaken, the PEG tube feeding becomes the patient's sole source of nutrition. Accordingly, it is essential to figure out which PEG delivery method the patient can best tolerate and to have the surgical procedure sooner rather than later in this journey.

*T*he PEG is a feeding tube that is placed (via a surgical procedure) directly into the stomach with an access point that rests outside the navel. Liquid food, nutritional supplements, and medications are injected into the PEG—completely bypassing the mouth and swallowing muscles. After initially nixing the idea of having a PEG put in, my mom, after consistent lobbying by her nonmedical team and, most effectively, by Dr. Robert, eventually changed her mind and agreed to the procedure in July 2013.

Our neurologist recommended two gastroenterologists to perform the PEG surgery. We were told that it was a relatively simple procedure and in many cases is done on an outpatient basis. At this point, my mom's speech was slurred (think of someone who has had at least two drinks more than usual), and when she called the first doctor's office, the nurse was very rude and gave my mom a difficult time. After that exchange, the first doctor was crossed off the list, and we reached out to the second doctor on the list, which in hindsight was truly a blessing. Of all the doctors that we encountered during this journey, Dr. Y---- was above and beyond the most engaged, caring, and proactive physician we came across. (The other notable positive experience was with an ER doctor at Cornell Medical Center.)

My mom's surgery seemed anything but ordinary. Instead of being released that afternoon or the next day, my mom spent five or six nights over the July 4 weekend in the hospital as swelling in the stomach area took some time to resolve. There was also some irritation at the surgical site. The excess bloating and irritation are all common occurrences. Fortunately, it was nothing too serious, but we did need to have Doctor Y---- reexamine the surgical site on several occasions.

With the PEG in place, the next part of the process was learning how to care and manage the PEG process. Initially, the PEG was meant to supplement typical mouth feedings, but over time as the swallowing/bulbar muscles weakened, the tube feeding became my mom's sole source of nutrition. During this transition, there was a constant struggle to reach the two-thousand-daily-calorie target. My mom tried keeping a food journal, but it was difficult to maintain and update. The food journal also proved to be a source of tension at certain times, as my mom's inability to meet the daily target was met with disappointment.

The overall care of the site and the flushing/cleaning protocol were relatively easy to learn. There was a distilled water flush both before and after the feedings. Learning the proper balance between continuous feeding (over a twelve-hour period) versus bolus feeding (ingesting the cans at mealtime) was the hard part. Suffice it to say, from July 2013 onward, feeling nauseous was the new norm for my mother. Whether it was trying to figure out the right balance of food and liquids (while my mom was still able to eat normally) or trying to find the right nutritional supplement with the proper caloric count, everything was trial and error, and it was a very frustrating process for everyone.

With continuous feeding, my mom was tethered to a pole that held a machine that pumped the liquid cans into the stomach through the PEG at a consistent rate throughout the day. These cycles usually took about twelve hours, so we tried to use the machine at night. The downside should be obvious; with the continuous liquids flowing into my mom's stomach at nighttime, she was forced to visit the bathroom numerous times during the ensuing hours. As a result, it was very difficult for my mom to get a solid night of sleep.

After growing frustrated with the continuous feeding option, we tried the bolus feeding. Here, the cans of liquid are directly injected into the feeding tube over a period of twenty to thirty minutes—essentially at mealtime. So this process occurred three to four times a day. This improved the overnight dislocation, but getting the required number of cans completed and managing the nausea was a puzzle that really was not solved until the last two weeks my mom was alive. At the suggestion of one of my mom's doctors, we even tried injecting decaffeinated coffee into the PEG roughly twenty minutes before each feeding to prepare the stomach for mealtime. The idea was that by stimulating the stomach before injecting the feeding cans, the stomach would be alerted that a meal was on its way and better able to digest the food. Unfortunately, this did not really reduce the nausea. For my mom, it turned out that using the gravity of the syringe to moderate the rate of the liquid flow into the PEG tube provided the least discomfort and nausea.

With the PEG in place and nausea the new normal, my mom struggled to get enough rest and to maintain her weight. With the nausea came additional discomforts, including constipation and becoming impacted. These were conditions that needed to be monitored and not allowed to linger without medical intervention. We were fortunate because anytime my mom's health really seemed to go off the rails, we were able to call Dr. Robert in California, who flagged when we needed to make a doctor's appointment or take my mom to the hospital. If you don't have a Dr. Robert in your family, then you must notify the doctor or clinic that you are working with as soon as any of these issues are present. Don't be shy or feel embarrassed about reaching out to your doctor or clinic to answer your questions. Remember, you are your patient's advocate, and I can assure you that no one in the medical establishment will be as vigilant or thoughtful about the care of your loved one as you will be.

Five

ROUTINES AND RITUALS

Given the numerous trips to the hospital, emergency room, and other medical appointments that this journey will take you on, it's important that your family maintain a master list of the patient's doctors as well as all of the patient's medication.

Like the PEG, over time, the BiPap machine will become the patient's sole source of noninvasive ventilation (before the tracheostomy tube procedure). While the BiPap machine helps with a patient's energy level and breathing function, most importantly, it helps remove carbon dioxide from a patient's body. Remember, carbon dioxide retention can kill a patient.

Keeping a normal routine is very important in the beginning. My mom continued to do her Pilates, play cards with her friends, and participate as much as her energy allowed. ALS does not impact the mind, so my mom was aware of all the bodily changes occurring in real time. That's one of the true tragedies of the disease. The patient is fully aware as her body shuts down and her mind becomes trapped in a listless mass.

Our medical routine consisted of monthly neurologist meetings with Dr. X---- (from Cornell) and quarterly clinic visits up at Columbia. At all of these meetings, some combination of Roy, me, my brother, Cyndee, Dr. Robert, my wife, or my sister-in-law attended and took notes to relay the commentary to those who could not attend.

One thing that proved very helpful was that we kept a master list of all of mom's doctors (neurologist, gastroenterologist, ENT) as well as a master list of all the medications that my mom was taking. The medications included Rilutek, various antinausea medications, and some antidepressants. The medical list was important anytime we visited a hospital or emergency room, as we provided the list to the attending physician at the time of examination. We found several benefits to maintaining a medical list. First, because my mom was nonverbal, the medical list helped answer many of the preadmission questions nurses and doctors typically ask during the examination. Second, the list helped protect against administering the wrong dosage of certain medications. Third, the list helped avoid prescribing medications that could cause an adverse reaction with my mom's existing medication.

As our journey progressed, different types of machines were ordered to help my mom maintain her strength and feel better. As mentioned previously, the BiPap machine is one of the most important machines. This is not a comfortable machine to use, and my mom did not embrace this machine initially. If your loved one is like my mom, you (or another member of the caregiving team) will initially get a lot of push back against utilizing the BiPap machine. Resist all temptation to placate the patient. Coax, cajole, bribe, and do whatever it takes to get your loved one using the machine as soon as possible—it's literally a matter of life or death!

As the ALS progressed and my mom's breathing became shallower and shallower (and she became weaker and weaker), she was more receptive to using the BiPap and finally did use the machine on a consistent basis. As highlighted earlier, the BiPap needs to be embraced by the patient at the earliest possible time—even if it's uncomfortable and takes multiple attempts to get the setting just right (Through trial and error, a respiratory therapist tries to find the proper setting, which can be adjusted over time).

It is important to understand from the start of the ALS journey that the BiPap machine, over time, becomes the primary source of ventilation for the patient and is the final stage of ventilation before the tracheostomy and mechanical ventilator—much in the same way that the PEG eventually becomes the sole source of feeding and nutrition. A cough assist machine and suction machine (to help a patient remove the phlegm in her chest) were also recommended to us.

A patient and a patient's family can refer to various sources to learn about the disease and how to help protect and improve a patient's immediate surroundings. The Muscular Dystrophy Association (MDA) provides an in-home evaluation to suggest how to protect the patient in the home setting, whether it's putting up guardrails, raising the height of the toilet seat, utilizing a shower seat, etc. Once a doctor writes the prescription, a home evaluation can be scheduled and coordinated through the local MDA chapter.

In terms of additional resources to aid in the care of a patient, it helps to understand the differences between a nurse's aide (NA), a licensed practical nurse (LPN), and a registered nurse (RN). An NA is really like a companion for the patient. The NA can help with walking, washing, bathing, and basically all nonmedical life functions, including going to the bathroom. The LPN can do everything that an NA can do but can also help administer medicines and is better trained to help monitor a patient's overall health. An RN can do everything that a NA or LPN can do but is more skilled and has the most medical training and education.

There are different service providers that can help assist in coordinating the care of a patient. We were pleased with SeniorBridge as a service provider. Of all the medical service providers that we contacted, SeniorBridge was the only provider that met with our family in person to talk about our mother's condition and to help develop a plan of care for her. SeniorBridge was referred to me by an acquaintance whose father also had ALS.

Interestingly, we were not allowed to interview the NA, LPN, or RN before they came to the hospital or to our home to provide care to my mother.

We provided feedback to SeniorBridge after the work shift was completed. My mom felt comfortable with some nurses and not with others. The other medical service providers did not offer face-to-face meetings. These providers just wanted us to select the type of help we needed (NA, LPN, or RN) from a roster of health-care workers on staff. It goes without saying that an NA, LPN, or RN that has already worked with an ALS patient is preferable to someone who has not.

Understanding the insurance labyrinth can be quite an overwhelming process. My mom had both long-term care insurance and Medicare insurance. For the long-term care insurance, it's important to reach out to the provider and understand the lay of the land sooner rather than later in the journey. Some policies have a ninety-day activation period, and other policies start right away. It's essential to understand what type of policy a patient has in order to properly plan for his or her care. On the Medicare side, each hospital stay allowed us to interact with a social worker who explained what type of coverage my mom was entitled to under the Medicare program. Again, it was a cumbersome labyrinth to navigate.

With ALS, it is quite likely that your loved one will be in the hospital on at least several occasions. In addition to always having access to your master doctor and medication lists, it is critical to know who has the patient's health-care proxy and who, if anyone, is the patient's power of attorney.

Six

The ALS "Talk"

I am not sure that there ever is a right time to talk about death, end-of-life decisions, and burial desires. Based on our family's experience, I think ripping the Band-Aid off and having those difficult conversations sooner rather than later is the best approach to addressing these questions, because not getting to have these conversations is likely far worse than having them at what may be perceived to be an inappropriate time.

There is never an easy time to talk about death and dying with your children. Our family dynamic was unique; we spent a lot of time together across the generational divide. My mom was very involved in her grandchildren's lives; she attended school plays, sporting events, birthday parties, camp visiting days, etc. She was active and present. We all shared a summer home together, so the grandkids had observed a decline in my mom's physical activity, the loss of weight, and the slurred speech. Her slurred speech seemed to be most observed by her grandchildren. As a result, we discussed my mom's illness at a relatively early stage when she had to have PEG placement surgery. We explained to our children the following points:

1. Mima (as my mom was called by her grandchildren) had a medical condition/disease, and the doctors were trying to help her feel better. We consciously avoided saying that Mima was sick, because everyone gets sick and usually he or she gets better;
2. Mima's condition/disease was not contagious, and no one could catch her illness.
3. No one did anything to cause or bring about Mima's medical condition/disease.

I was amazed at how all the grandkids responded and adapted to our new normal. The slurred speech, the PEG feeding, the lower energy—all were accepted. The grandkids thought that the BiPap machine was cool (and several wanted to try it on), and the PEG feeding was amazing to watch. (To think that food could go directly into the stomach and bypass swallowing was a concept that took some time for the grandkids to fully grasp.)

Along the way, we tried to provide "bread crumbs" for the kids that Mima was not getting better. For my family, it really hit home when Mima could not go up to grandparents' visiting day at sleep-away camp. I think that my sons (ages nine and seven at the time), in their own way, began to grasp that Mima's health was descending. Since Mima had enthusiastically attended grandparents' day for my oldest son during his first summer of sleep-away camp, I had to explain her absence the second and third summers. The second summer I explained to the boys (now that my second son was also attending the same camp) that Mima needed some surgery to try to help manage her condition. During the second summer visiting day, each boy sent video messages back to Mima. By the third summer (July 2014), I believe the boys understood that Mima was not strong enough to attend visiting day and did not seem to be getting better. I explained that Mima was too weak to travel and that she was trying to get stronger so that she could make it down to Jamaica over Christmas.

The Journey

As the final weeks approached, we called a family meeting to let the kids know that Mima was not getting better and that she was not going to get better. The subtlety of the message escaped my two younger children, but my older son (age ten) understood the message, and it hit him hard. He was the first grandchild in our family and very close to my mother. It was a sad night, and we made ourselves available to answer any questions that any of the children had about Mima. We also alerted the children's schools about what was going on with our family, so they could keep an eye out for our children. We let each school know that my mom would be in hospice care within the month.

There is never really an easy time to talk to a parent about dying regardless of whether he or she has a terminal disease or not. My brother and I were very close to my mom. Yet, despite our closeness, talking about death was an awkward conversation. We needed to confirm how my mom wanted to be buried or cremated, what type of ceremony she wanted, and to make sure that all of her affairs were in order. We were fortunate because, during one of Cyndee's visits to see my mom, she was able to start the dialogue. We all kind of knew that my mom wanted to be cremated (like my father) but we needed to confirm it.

When my mom wanted to talk about these issues after she was first diagnosed with ALS, I wanted to avoid the conversation because I thought that we had a lot of time and did not want to dwell on the negatives. At the end, when it was time to have those conversations, I was hesitant because I did not want to convey to my mom that I thought that the end was near. I did not want her to give up. Needless to say, there is no right time to talk about these issues, so I think ripping the Band-Aid off is the best approach. Not getting to have these conversations is likely far worse than having them at what may be perceived to be an inappropriate time. I am not sure that there ever is a right time. These conversations are important, especially when considering end-of-life discussions like a do not resuscitate (DNR), extraordinary measures, and the "trache". My brother and I were my mom's healthcare proxies, and we needed to have these discussions.

Seven

The Progression of ALS: What to Expect

Two landmines threw my family for a loop when they exploded. One was a medical condition called hyponatremia, and the other was dangerously elevated carbon dioxide levels. Both landmines put my mom back in the emergency room and eventually back in the hospital for multi-night stays.

⌣⟶

As a nonmedical person, it was amazing to watch the progression of the disease. ALS is deliberate, relentless, and ruthless. In the eight months after my mom's PEG surgery, my mom fully lost her ability to speak, she shed another twenty pounds, and she became reliant on the PEG as her sole nutritional source. Post PEG surgery, my mom's nausea became a steady state of being—the new norm. Between normal mouth feedings and using the nutritional cans through the PEG, my mom's stomach never seemed to be settled. The unsettled stomach and constant state of nausea led to continuous trips to the bathroom, which inevitably impacted her ability to get a good night's sleep. The lack of solid sleep led to increased fatigue and decreased energy. Everything sort of snowballed and, at the end, seemed to catch us all off guard.

We were ill prepared for two very scary events in the last month of my mom's life, and I hope they will be on other families' radar screens in the future. My daughter celebrated her fifth birthday at the end of the summer of 2014. My mom rallied to attend the party and to celebrate my daughter's birthday outside with friends. This was only the second time all summer that my mom had attended a social event—the other being her birthday in June. Other than that, my mom slowly withdrew from social activities and spent most of her time in her bedroom.

During the 2014 summer, the ALS Ice Bucket Challenge (the Challenge) garnered a lot of attention. The Challenge helped both raise awareness of the disease and increase donations to various ALS charities. While some discussion about the disease is better than no discussion, to me, the discourse seemed a bit on the superficial side. It seemed that most people talking about ALS still did not fully appreciate how deadly and aggressive the disease was.

Two episodes in particular really hit home for me during this period. The first occurred at work, and the other occurred on my phone. At work, the Challenge initiated a discussion in my office about ALS. I recall debating whether to join the discussion and correct some of the misinformation being bandied about or to just sit this one out. Since only a few people at work knew of my mom's condition, I decided to stay out of the conversation. In retrospect, I feel like I wasted an opportunity to inform.

The other event occurred in mid-August when my wife sent a video clip to my phone. The video showed my three children, ages four to ten, taking the Challenge. Watching the video brought tears to my eyes, as I knew how personal this was for our family.

Recently, when my daughter and I were looking through the pictures from her fifth birthday party, she commented that Mima was not smiling in any of the pictures. At this point in the journey, my mom had lost the ability to control her facial muscles. Over the two weeks after my daughter's party at the end of August, my mom's health descended several steps. During conversations with her, she seemed to "check out" or "space out" midconversation while we were talking to her or when she was typing and responding. These events became more frequent and unpredictable. She also became much more tired and fatigued—rarely getting out of her bed or sitting chair. Her breathing became shallower, and she was up all night, in and out of the bathroom. To protect against an accident, my mom was now wearing adult diapers. It was as if a switch had been turned on to a new, meaningfully lower level of health.

When we described my mom's condition to my uncle in California, he was surprised by the rapid decline and recommended that my mom get her blood worked up as soon as possible, because he felt that something did not make sense. We reached out to Dr. Y----and coordinated the blood test for the next day. When the bloodwork came back, it showed that my mom had a condition called hyponatremia, which is a low level of sodium in the blood. In severe cases, hyponatremia can lead to a coma and be fatal. My mom needed to be admitted to the hospital immediately, so they could raise her sodium count back to a healthy level. Given her compromised breathing and weak swallowing muscles, her body was retaining more water than usual, which had caused her sodium level to decline.

At this time, my mom was nonverbal, so communicating with the medical staff was obviously challenging. Again, we had our master doctor list and medicine list with us, which reduced a lot of the medical bottleneck during admission and conversations with the doctors. Our in-hospital experience was mixed; some on the medical team actually read her medical chart and understood that she could still communicate by writing and that her mental faculties were still intact. Others would come into the room, speak to her, and wait for her to respond until a family member notified them that Mom was nonverbal. Interestingly, some interpreted my mom's nonverbal status as being deaf and would suddenly start raising their voices and enunciating their speech in an exaggerated, loud voice. My mom would shoot us a look that screamed, "Someone please tell this doctor that I am not deaf!"

In our family, we each took turns staying with my mom overnight since that was the most difficult time for her, a nonverbal patient, to communicate with the nursing staff. Again, our experience with the nurses was mixed. Some were engaging, nurturing, and warm while others were just punching a time card. And when we could not stay overnight, we made sure that an NA was with her to help her at night and to reach out to the nurses if need be.

This first trip to the ER resulted in a five-night stay at the hospital. My mom was released on Thursday, September 11, 2014. Naively, our family thought that once the doctors were able to raise her sodium levels back to a normal range, my mom would regain the medical status she had at my daughter's birthday party before this multiple step-down decline in her health. While hope springs eternal, the reality is that ALS does not pause, and there is no going backward and recapturing lost time or improved health. That is why it's so important to be aggressive at the beginning of the diagnosis.

If you are the patient, take in all the calories you can (if you don't like eating ice cream, too bad), use all the recommended breathing machines, and try to maintain as much of a normal routine as possible. If the patient is someone you love, be diligent and focused on making sure he or she consumes as many calories as possible. In our case, it was difficult for family members to get my mom to stick to the calorie plan and to utilize the BiPap machine. In retrospect, what we needed was an unaffiliated individual to monitor and oversee my mom's regiment (to the extent she would have permitted that).

After the hyponatremia episode, we were more keenly aware to look out for the subtle changes in my mom's health. Was she as responsive? How was her breathing? Was she out of it or still engaged? My wife purchased a finger-pulse oximeter to monitor my mom's oxygen level. If her pulse oxygen reading dropped below ninety, we knew that such a decline could be an issue and that my mom might need an oxygen supplement.

What we so clearly did not fully appreciate was that my mom's oxygen level was only one side of an important two-sided coin. The other side of the coin is that the carbon dioxide level is not readily testable, yet it is a major risk that every ALS family should know about. Basically, when a person inhales, the lungs bring in clean oxygen to the body, and when a person exhales, the lungs release the carbon dioxide from the body. As my mom's breathing became more compromised, the exhale part really sneaked up on all of us. My mom's inability to expel the carbon dioxide led to a dangerously high buildup of carbon dioxide in her system. In a healthy person, a normal level of carbon dioxide might be forty. In my mom's case, her carbon dioxide level steadily rose over the course of her illness—sometimes into the seventy-to-eighty range.

As I mentioned earlier, my mom was released from the hospital on September 11, 2014, which was a Thursday. She was feeling OK—everything being relative. She returned home, and we watched her carefully. Two days later, on Saturday at midday September 13, 2014, both Roy and my brother observed that her health again started to decline. Her pulse oxygen reading dipped into the mideighties on one hand (each hand provided a different oxygen-level reading, but both showed a level well below ninety). We put the BiPap machine on her to try to improve her breathing. Initially this worked, but soon after my mom's oxygen level started to show consistently lower results, and her ability to focus declined. We called her pulmonary doctor first (who had also been her primary care physician for the last fifteen years). You are only first hearing about him at this point in the disease's progression because he was essentially absent from my mom's medical care up until the "final out of the final inning" of her life. He was a total and complete disappointment! I hope that you will not have such a disappointment. He is referred to as the "phantom pulmonologist" throughout the remainder of this book. Not surprisingly, he was unreachable, and the doctor covering for him suggested either ordering oxygen for my mom or taking my mom back to the hospital. The thought of returning to the hospital was not a choice that excited anyone in our family, as we realized that there was a high probability my mom would not make it out of the hospital.

Once again, we reached out to Dr. Robert in California to get his medical advice. It was clear in his mind that if Mom's numbers did not respond to the BiPap usage and her physical condition did not improve, we had to take her back to the hospital—no ifs, ands, or buts. Despite hoping that my mom would respond to the BiPap machine, her condition did not improve, and we prepared to take her back to the hospital. We called 911, explained that my mom was having difficulty breathing and that we needed to go to the ER.

We alerted the doorman to expect an ambulance and paramedics. After we hung up the phone, we repacked my mom's hospital bag, gathered her medical and doctor list, and waited. We called my uncle in California to let him know we were headed back to the hospital and suggested that it was a good idea for Cyndee to come back to New York to be with us.

As we soon learned, when a 911 call goes out, the first responders are typically the Fire Department of New York (FDNY). After several minutes, two FDNY officers were on the scene. Professional, thorough, and caring, they took my mom's information and explained that they typically respond before the paramedics because they tend to be in more areas than the ambulances. They took my mom's vital signs and tried to comfort her. Shortly thereafter, the paramedics arrived. We went through the same process, and they provided her with nasal oxygen. As my mom breathed in the oxygen, her demeanor and skin color improved; she became more responsive. The paramedics prepared to transport her back to the hospital.

Several minutes later, the New York Police Department officers (NYPD) arrived. As New York's finest explained, when paramedics are dispatched to a home, the police usually accompany them to make sure that the domestic situation is safe and secure.

My mom, Roy, my brother, and I all climbed into the back of the ambulance. My brother and I called our respective wives and let them know that we were heading back to the hospital. As my mom took in the oxygen, the color started to return to her face, and her awareness significantly improved—everything being relative. When we arrived at the ER, we were wheeled into one of the ER holding pods and seen by several ER doctors. My mom's condition was far from stable, and after several doctors asked whether we had discussed putting in a "trache", it became clear to all of us that my mom's health had taken yet another step-down.

That day, I learned many things about the different types of blood tests. The ER doctors now needed to draw blood from an artery instead of just a vein. This type of blood test is slightly more painful, but it provides the most accurate view of a patient's blood characteristics, because the blood is the freshest coming right out of the heart. As is the case in hospital settings, you see medical students, medical residents, and medical chiefs. No one ever left my mom alone, and when the ER attendant wanted to draw blood from my mom's artery, he tried to talk a medical resident through the process. After watching this young medical student prod my mom several times, I suggested that the doctor perform the blood test himself. He skillfully drew the blood from the artery on his first attempt. Over the next several hours, we were visited by various medical teams who examined and met my mom. Her condition eventually stabilized at this lower level of health.

It was around 10:00 p.m. or 11:00 p.m. when we met with the full medical team who said that they would admit my mother. We were all circled around my mom's hospital bed, listening intensely to what the doctors were saying and asking many questions. Right in the middle of this meeting, my mom's sister, Cyndee, arrived from California like a whirling dervish. Obviously strained from the cross-country trip and my mom's failing health, she demanded to know what was going on. Her question offered a comedic pause in what was a tense moment.

After catching our breaths and introducing Cyndee to the medical team, we continued the meeting. It was clear from this all-hands-on-deck meeting that the ALS was now meaningfully impacting my mom's diaphragm muscle and that she was approaching respiratory failure. It was a long night that started in the ER at around 5:00 p.m., and we were finally admitted into a room at roughly 2:00 a.m. Since we all recognized that we were going to be spending a lot more time in the hospital, we divided our resources as Roy and Cyndee went home, and I, our nurse, and my brother stayed with my mom until she reached her room.

With my mom back in the hospital for the second time in two weeks, we made sure that she had twenty-four-hours a day nurse care. Being in a hospital and being nonverbal is not a great combination. The hospital staff was responsive and worked closely with the nurses that we hired to make sure that my mom had the necessary coverage. We were visited by both new doctors and some familiar ones. The diagnosing neurologist visited, if not daily, then every other day. A bit distant and somewhat aloof, he confirmed to my brother and me what we had already surmised: my mom's health was nearing an end.

The "trache" conversation was no longer in the background but was now front and center. As the ER doctors had highlighted during our recent visit, we needed to answer this question sooner rather than later. As several doctors explained to our family, the "trache" surgery is a relatively routine procedure that requires general anesthesia. In layman's terms, a trachea tube is placed in a patient's windpipe to allow air to reach the lungs. A ventilation machine is then attached to the tube, takes over, and provides all the inhaling and exhaling that a patient needs. In essence, it completely replaces the function of the diaphragm muscle. When we chatted with the different doctors, it was clear that, typically, patients get worse before they get better postsurgery and that it takes a patient two to three weeks to acclimate to the "trache" in the hospital.

It's important to recognize that at this point, my mom's health was already meaningfully compromised. My mom was largely confined to her hospital bed, needed help walking, and exercise or "getting up and around" now consisted of just trying to sit up in a chair for a period of time, usually thirty to forty-five minutes. Physical trips to the bathroom became less frequent and then nonexistent—the bedpan became my mom's bathroom. My mom spent three quarters of the day on the BiPap machine, and when she was off the machine, her condition declined, and she got noticeably weaker. The doctors agreed; as each day passed, her usage of the BiPap machine would increase, and ultimately she would need to be on it twenty-four hours a day.

My mom's view on the "trache" evolved during her illness. Early in her illness, my mom made it clear to me and my brother that she did not want to live on a ventilator; she provided a DNR and did not want any extraordinary measures used on her. However, in September 2014, my mom's view on this topic changed. Our family learned of this change during my mom's first hospital stay for hyponatremia. My mom indicated to both my brother and the neurologist that she wanted to have a "trache" put in. I was surprised. I later confirmed her wishes with my brother and again when she was readmitted to the hospital for the breathing difficulty. Despite having her health-care proxy, if it was her wish to have the procedure, then we would honor her desire and have the "trache" procedure.

During this time, we also received word from the "phantom pulmonologist" that he wanted to meet with the family to discuss my mother's health. My mom's phantom pulmonologist always seemed to make the rounds and visit my mom when no family member was around. My brother, Roy, Cyndee, and I all met at the phantom pulmonologist's office on the morning of September 16, 2014. While my brother and I had my mom's health-care proxy, it was important for all of us to be together at this meeting to all hear the same comments and have the opportunity to each ask questions.

It was a very awkward, strange meeting as the phantom pulmonologist and his physician partner informed us that my mom was experiencing respiratory failure caused by the ALS as the disease had now progressed to my mom's breathing muscles. I suppose each doctor has his or her own unique method for delivering negative or sad news. At various times during the conversation it almost seemed that the doctor was smiling, which I believe was some sort of nervous response triggered by the subject of conversation. I found one exchange particularly curious. I explained to the doctor that we, as a family, typically go away in December, and I asked whether he thought that my mom would be able to go this year. He said, "That would take a lot of work." That still resonates with me. What a load of crap! There are a lot of things that would require "a lot of work" to improve—reversing or halting respiratory failure does not seem to be one of them. ALS does not go in reverse! Why not just say, "your mom will not be in any condition to travel"?

Regardless of this exchange, the key points were that my mom was going into respiratory failure and that it was a question of *when* and not *whether* we needed to decide to go forward with the tracheostomy. If we elected not to put in the "trache", then my mom would likely get pneumonia and/or go into cardiac arrest. Neither path was particularly attractive. He informed us that an ENT doctor performs the surgery. After we left the doctor, we went out to lunch and talked about the doctor meeting and how and who would bring my mom up to speed on what the phantom pulmonologist had to say.

Needless to say, not every family member thought that the "trache" was a good idea. Three out of the four of us thought that the "trache" made sense. The dissenting voter reasoned that given my mom's current physical condition and rapidly declining quality of health, how much worse would she get by the time we decided to have the procedure, and what did my mom's health and quality of life look like on the other side of the operation? Would my mom really want to live that way? It was an open and honest conversation where everyone's voice was listened to and respected. At the end of the lunch, we all agreed to support whatever decision my mom made despite some of our individual misgivings.

As the oldest son, I was chosen to deliver the summary of the doctor's meeting in a neutral, unalarming, and fully disclosed manner (as much as my personality would permit). It was a very difficult conversation. I explained matter-of-factly that the disease had spread into her breathing muscles, that she would need to spend more and more time on the BiPap machine, and that the next decision to be made was whether to have the "trache" procedure.

My mom and I were very close, and I have no doubt that she could read the expression on my face and the emotion in my body language. I asked her if she understood, and she nodded. During this time, Cyndee vacillated between being a "trache" proponent and not wanting my mom to suffer anymore. Despite all of the sadness and upheaval, our family rallied together. The grandkids visited my mom in the hospital, and my wife even coordinated for my mom to have a mani-pedi in her hospital room. My mom was always a lady.

Later that night, I sat with my mom and told her that she needed to make the "trache" decision based on what she wanted to do and not on what she thought I, my brother, or her sister wanted her to do; she needed to make *this* decision based on how she wanted to live. My mom had spent her life always looking out and protecting my brother and me. I told her that she had done an amazing job and that she did not need to look out for my brother or me in the same way anymore. She needed to focus on looking out for herself and making the decision on how she wanted to live—and ultimately pass away. When I finished talking, she nodded and tapped her heart and pointed to me. That was her way of saying, "I love you."

On Wednesday, September 17, 2014, my mom decided that she wanted to wait a little while before making the "trache" decision. At this point in my mom's care, there was nothing going on in the hospital setting that could not be provided in the home setting. The hospital was going to discharge her that afternoon. Given how hospital bureaucracies work, the afternoon discharge turned into the early evening and then into the late evening. We decided to stay the night and leave the first thing in the morning. This decision to stay the night caused a bit of a commotion in the hospital, but we argued that discharging her in the middle of the night made very little sense, and various care providers, both on and off the record, felt that we should stay the night as well.

Once we made the decision to stay the night, my mom seemed relieved. She asked if her sister would spend the night with her in the hospital. Without hesitation, Cyndee readily agreed. I considered this an ominous request. When my father passed away over twenty years ago, I vividly recall him asking me to spend the night with him the night before he passed away. I wondered whether my mom thought that she was going to pass away that night. The night was another restless, energy-draining evening as my mom became more and more dependent on the BiPap. She was discharged from the hospital that Thursday morning, September 18, 2014.

In the ambulance, heading back to her apartment, with Cyndee, my sister-in-law, and Roy, my mom informed Cyndee (in writing) that she did not want to go back to the hospital under any circumstances and that she did not want to have the "trache" procedure. She had reached her breaking point; enough was enough. When this was relayed to me, I had mixed emotions. On the one hand, I was so profoundly sad that the end was fast approaching, but on the other hand, I was relieved that my mom decided not to put herself through another surgery and the attendant risks involved with the "trache" procedure. She had endured so much already.

I left work and met my brother to go see my mom and to hear or read for myself that she did not want to go back to the hospital. When we arrived at my mom's apartment, she asked (in writing) if we had spoken to Cyndee and understood her wishes. I told her that her sister had relayed the message, but we wanted to hear directly from her as well, which she clearly confirmed. At this point, life had come full circle as the progression of the disease had rendered my mom incapable of eating, bathing, washing, or going to the bathroom without assistance. For all intents and purposes, physically, my mom was an infant again, while mentally she had to endure this regression. We entered the final phase of this journey with hospice care.

Eight

Hospice Care

For the first time since this awful journey started, our family collectively felt after meeting with the hospice care provider that some entity (doctor, service provider, and clinic) was finally in control, focused, and truly coordinating all of my mom's medical needs.

⌒

With my mom finally settled at home, we scheduled a meeting on Friday, September 19, 2014, with the Metropolitan Jewish Health System (MJHS) hospice care service. The discharging hospital social worker recommended MJHS to our family, as MJHS had prior experience working with our home health-care service provider (SeniorBridge). Hospice care, palliative care, or end-of-life care typically is the lead service provider when a patient has less than six months to live. Our family was fortunate to work with MJHS.

On Friday morning, we met the hospice care representative and reviewed the services, procedures, and mechanics of the care. The representative, a registered nurse, was warm, compassionate, and informative. After the several-hour interview and patient-care review, my brother, Cyndee, Roy, and I all breathed a collective sigh of relief. For the first time since this awful journey started, we felt that some entity (doctor, service provider, and clinic) was in control, focused, and truly coordinating all of my mom's medical needs.

As discussed earlier in the day, that night my mom was visited by a coordinating nurse, staffed with a qualified overnight nurse, and delivered a cough assist machine and suction machine. These machines were not my mom's favorite by any stretch of the imagination. However, in the hospital, the doctors gave my mom a lidocaine spray before using the suctioning device, which seemed to ease my mom's discomfort. The issue was when we were discharged by the hospital, they did not give us the lidocaine spray to take home or provide a prescription to fill outside the hospital.

We reached out to the attending ER doctor who provided care to my mom, and he wrote us a prescription for the special spray. I remember going back to the hospital where he met me in the general reception area. It truly was one of the few positive, noteworthy medical experiences during this process. Armed with the prescription, our family was sent out on a frantic search for this mystery spray. Each family member called different pharmacies looking for it—no one had it, and no pharmacy could create it. Once again, we reached out to Dr. Robert, in California, who was able to find a compounding pharmacy to make the spray and send it back to New York. Unfortunately, the spray arrived the day after my mom passed away. Talk about total medical inefficiency—this was a frustrating exercise and one that I hope you will never have to go through.

On Friday night, our family coordinated for all six grandchildren to come over to Mima's house. Mima had a special gift for each of them. Each of the six grandchildren had an opportunity to spend some time with their Mima and most importantly, my mom was able to share their squeals of excitement as they each opened up their gifts. Most of us realized that this was going to be one of the last times that the grandkids would be able to spend time with their Mima. It was bittersweet. We all held back our tears as the kids excitedly opened their gifts and then gave a big hug to Mima to thank her.

The Journey

The hospice care was in place, and services started to flow. We felt for the first time that we were in front of this disease instead of always chasing it. After lengthy discussions with Cyndee about when she should go back to California and potential return timelines, we all felt that this was the window to go back. Saturday morning, my mom was resting, and the prior night was relatively uneventful. Not a lot of rest, but that was the norm. Cyndee communicated with my mom that morning, and they both agreed now was a good time for Cyndee to return to California to tend to her family and then return in a week after the Jewish holidays. Cyndee left that morning.

Saturday was largely uneventful. My mom rested, and we all took turns spending time with her. My wife took my sons to their flag football game, and she provided me real-time game updates. We each took turns running errands, picking up things to keep around the house from the various medical supply stores in the area. That afternoon, my brother and I communicated with my mom about the type of ceremony she wanted to have to celebrate her life. As expected, she confirmed that she wanted a memorial service like we had for my father at our home in California—no religious officials, just speeches commemorating her life.

At that point, we had confirmed all of the outstanding questions regarding the disposition of her body and what type of ceremony she wanted. I remember leaving my mom's apartment in the afternoon to go home and see my kids with the plan to return that evening. In the early evening, I went to get a haircut and then returned to my mom's apartment with my wife. That evening was also largely uneventful. My mom's condition did not show any material change from the already low engagement levels.

As I mentioned earlier, during this journey, I read and reread *Tuesdays with Morrie* several times. I found solace in those words and read certain passages from the book to my mom. When I went to say good night to her on that Saturday night, I read the following passages:

As long as we can love each other and remember the feeling of love we had, we can die without ever really going away. All the love you created is still there. All the memories are still there. You live on in the hearts of everyone you have touched and nurtured while you were here.

Death ends a life, not a relationship.[iii]

She tapped her heart and pointed to me afterward. I kissed her on the forehead and then walked home with my wife. Roy and the MJHS nurse remained at my mom's bedside.

Nine

My Mom's Passing

In retrospect, the timing of my mom passing away was quite amazing. My mom said good-bye to her sister, her grandkids, and then to all her children and daughters-in-law. My mom was ready—she had endured enough—and I believe she left on her own terms before the disease could do further destruction.

‿⁀

On the walk home from my mom's apartment, my wife expressed her sadness and frustration with my mom's current state of being. My wife felt that my mom was uncomfortable and would likely benefit from some pain medication (morphine). Up until that night, our family considered the morphine option the final leg of this journey and, rightfully or wrongfully, we believed that once we started the morphine drip there was no turning back, so we were hesitant to start the process too early. My wife said that she would not want to live like that if she were in my mom's shoes—I agreed. You may find, as I did, that it's easier to have that view as a third party as opposed to the afflicted person. We both agreed that the most important thing was for my mom not to suffer and to be comfortable and that we would revisit the morphine discussion in the next few days, depending on my mom's health. I suggested that nature would eventually run its course and that my mom just wanted to be comfortable and be in her home.

We were looking forward to going down to Philly the next day to see the Eagles football game. We ordered all the kids Eagles clothes to wear. When my phone rang that Saturday night (September 20, 2014) at 10:15 p.m., a few minutes after leaving my mom's side, I was surprised. My brother told me that the MJHS nurse had just called him and told him to come right back to the apartment. He then called me. I quickly put on my clothes and rushed over to my mom's apartment. I told my wife I would call her when I knew what was going on.

When I arrived and saw the facial expressions on Roy and my brother, I knew my mom had passed away. The nurse said that she took a big breath and then passed—no pain or distress. I texted my wife to let her know the news, and she came over to the apartment. The next few hours were a bit hectic and surreal as we started the burial process. We called a funeral home to request a pickup and started to sketch out the plans for her memorial service. I called Cyndee in California to tell her the news. She was devastated. Her pain was tangible. I called several of my mom's closest friends to tell them as well. I wanted to make sure that they heard the news from someone in our family as opposed to through the New York City gossip/yenta mill.

Even in the saddest of times, there are things that can make you smile or take your mind off the pain. You never know where they will come from, but they seem to appear often. For us, it was when the funeral home representative showed up at the apartment at around 1:30 a.m. to pick up my mom and take her to the funeral parlor. Right out of the HBO show *Six Feet Under*, the funeral representative appeared in a jet-black suit wearing thick black sports goggles (Kareem Abdul-Jabbar style) and accompanied by his female associate. It was such an interesting mixture of solemnness and activity—we mused whether this was his "game time," or whether the glasses were prescription—whatever it took to distract us from the current pain and sadness.

After my mom was taken to the funeral home, my wife and sister-in-law left, and my brother and I stayed at the apartment to make sure that we had a game plan for the next few days. We all acknowledged and dreaded how difficult the next morning was going to be when we had to tell our children that Mima had passed away. My brother and I thought that we should try to get all the kids together the next day after we told them about Mima so that they could be together, and we could start the planning process.

In retrospect, my mom's timing was quite amazing. She said good-bye to her sister, all her grandkids, and then to all her children and daughters-in-law. My mom was beyond exhausted—she'd endured enough—and I believe left on her own terms before the disease could do further destruction to her body and mind.

Sunday morning was one of the most emotional days of my life. Each of my three children woke up early, excited to go down to Philadelphia for the Eagles game. We never made it to the game. They dressed in their Eagles gear and checked their bags that they packed for the game. I told them that we had to have a family meeting, and I explained to them that Mima had died the night before. Many tears were shed. My middle son came to my side to comfort me as I told them that Mima had passed away. Because we shared so many family events, trips, and homes together, I told our children that if they wanted to see Mima, they should close their eyes and think about the different events that they had shared together. That way, Mima would still be here with them, and her memory would always live on inside each of them. My brother and I brought our families together later that morning so that they could talk about Mima and be with one another. The six grandkids/cousins ranged in age from three to ten. Being together seemed to comfort them. While they were together, my brother, Roy, and I met at the funeral home to start the memorial process.

Ten

The Memorial Service

At the memorial service (September 23, 2014), we celebrated my mom's extraordinary life. People who did not know my mom well or had never met her came up to my brother and me after the memorial and said that after listening to the service they felt that they "knew" my mom and how lucky we were to have someone like that so central in our lives.

⌣⌐

We met with a very thoughtful, compassionate funeral director at the local funeral parlor. We needed to answer a bunch of different questions regarding my mom—some of which we knew the answers to while others we did not. We conferenced-in Cyndee to fill in the information gaps and to work out the timing of my mom's service. We had one of those awkward funny moments when we were considering the timing of how and when my mom would be cremated. We were especially sensitive to Cyndee's desire to say good-bye to my mom. Cyndee had returned to California the same day my mom passed, and we wanted to see if she wanted to come back to New York to say good-bye to her in person or whether we should proceed with the cremation within the typically prescribed time—usually within forty-eight to seventy-two hours. After going back and forth on several timing options, I suggested that Cyndee could FaceTime my mom, and I would put the phone in her resting casket so that Cyndee could see my mom and tell her all the things that she wanted to say. We all nervously laughed and decided to put Cyndee on the speakerphone for her to say good-bye to her sister instead.

The other curious moment occurred when we chose the casket for my mom to be transported in to the crematorium. The funeral director showed us three different options to purchase: a low-end casket, a medium-end casket, and a high-end casket. There was a price spread of several thousand dollars between the low-end casket and high-end models. I thought that caskets were purchased when someone is buried, not cremated—I was wrong. This struck me as odd. Why would we need to purchase a casket that would be incinerated within the next forty-eight hours? I still don't have a good answer to that question, but that's how the cremation business works.

Later that evening, I explained to our children that we were going to have a memorial service to honor and celebrate Mima and that if they wanted to speak at the service, they could. No pressure. Either way was fine—whatever each of them felt comfortable with was what they should do. I told them that I was going to speak, as were several other close family friends and family members. I also told them that they could write a note to Mima and that I would read it for them if they decided not to speak. I left it in their hands, and over the next few days, each of them wrote out a special note to Mima.

My mom was not a religious person, so it was not a surprise to us or her close friends that she did not want to have a religious figure officiate at her memorial service. My brother and I, along with help from our wives and Roy, organized the memorial service. My brother and I officiated the service and introduced each of the speakers that day.

When we arrived at the funeral chapel, I had another one of those awkward exchanges that still resonates with me. I showed all the kids where they were going to sit and from where they were going to speak. My mom was in her urn surrounded by two beautiful flower arrangements. My youngest child, a daughter, was very close to my mother. I showed her Mima's urn; She looked

46

at it and then back to me and asked "where was Mima, and how did she get into the urn?" I was caught off guard by the question. I thought about it for a moment, and then explained that Mima was in heaven, that Mima chose to have her body go to a special place where it was very hot, that the heat turned her body into sand, and the sand was placed in the urn—as opposed to being buried and placed in the ground. I thought it seemed like a reasonable explanation. Apparently not, because my daughter then asked, "But where is the rest of Mima, and how did she fit into that little thing?"

I was taken aback—I hoped that someone would come into the chapel and give me a reprieve from this conversation. No one came in, and I remained locked in mental hand-to-hand combat with my five-year-old daughter. Eventually, I was able to convey that all of Mima's body was made into very fine small grains of sand to fit into the urn and that Mima would now be next to my dad who was also cremated. After that exchange, I could not wait for the memorial service to begin.

At the memorial, two of my mom's closest friends spoke, as did her nieces, her brother-in-law, Roy, her grandchildren (five out of six of them), my sister-in-law, my brother, and me. At the memorial service, I said of Roy, "My mom was so lucky to have you in her life. There are no words that can express how well you cared for my mom both during the good times, as well as when things got challenging, and we are so appreciative of your efforts and love for her."

What was particularly comforting was that people who did not know my mom well or had never met her came up to my brother and me after the memorial and said that after listening to the service, they felt that they "knew" my mom and how lucky we were to have someone like that so central in our lives. We hosted people who wanted to show their respect at my mom's apartment over the next two days. It was a long process, but we as a family took comfort from the outpouring of love and support.

Eleven

WHAT WE LEARNED FROM THIS JOURNEY

There were many lessons that we learned during this journey. We learned the importance of family, as working together and supporting one another were critical. In retrospect, what we really needed was an independent third-party health-care supervisor who could oversee and manage my mom's caloric intake and breathing machine utilization. Each family member was only able to accomplish so much as my mom was very strong-willed and determined to manage the illness on her own terms.

In retrospect, I wish we had done some things differently, and I wish we had been better prepared for other things that could have made this journey somewhat less painful and chaotic. Below is a list of those items that I hope will help other families dealing with ALS:

- I wish that we had shared our experience more publicly with our friends and acquaintances, because you never know who has gone through a similar experience or who might know someone who has gone through a similar experience. Hopefully, this book will prove to be a resource for others just starting this journey.

- I found the clinical setting to be impersonal and sterile, and I preferred the more personal and accessible monthly doctor visits. In the clinical setting, there was no one quarterbacking my mom's care. I felt as if we were on a rudderless ship that would get boarded and inspected and then left back out in the ocean after our quarterly exam was completed. The truth is that neither path is ideal, so pursuing parallel paths seemed to make the most sense for our family. Since there is a very limited medical playbook to combat this disease, the onus falls on us, the family members, to make sure that the patient takes in all the calories possible and utilizes the BiPap machine as much as possible.

- It's important to keep, maintain, and have readily accessible a master list of all the doctors and medicines that the patient is taking.

- The PEG is essential. Do not delay having this procedure, especially if you or your loved one has PBP or bulbar ALS. Take in as many calories as possible, and if that means embracing the PEG sooner rather than later, then so be it. Take the time to learn what works best for the individual patient. Over time, the PEG will be the patient's sole nutritional source. Losing weight accelerates a patient's medical descent as the body eventually starts to burn up muscle to feed itself. And the cycle of fatigue gets worse and worse.

- The BiPap machine is essential—do not wait too long before embracing this aid. The BiPap machine is critical because it takes the carbon dioxide out of the patient's body. As mentioned earlier, plain and simple—carbon dioxide retention can kill a patient.

- Calories, calories, calories—tell the patient to forget about his or her waistline and indulge.

- Understand a patient's insurance profile: long-term care policy, Medicare, etc.

- Understand who has the patient's health-care proxy.

- Understand who has the patient's power of attorney.

- Understand the patient's end-of-life decisions and burial wishes.
- Be on the lookout for hyponatremia, which is a low level of sodium in the blood. In severe cases, hyponatremia can lead to a coma and be fatal.
- Work closely with your family members and close friends. You are all on the same team, and everyone will need to help in some way, shape, or form (physically, emotionally, and/or financially).

Twelve

My Mom's Legacy Continues

My mom was the glue that held our family together. Her passion and focus were her family; she derived great joy from sharing and participating in all of our lives. The home that she built for our family to spend time together in was crafted and designed to make sure that everyone had their own living spaces and that each grandchild would be happy there.

We continue to honor my mother's legacy. We celebrated Thanksgiving together at the house that she built for the family, which my family continues to share with my brother's family. Moreover, we continued our family tradition and returned to Jamaica this past holiday season. My brother's family, my family, and Roy all revisited the same holiday spot that my mom so enjoyed with her children, boyfriend, and grandchildren. While the sense of loss was evident, we took comfort in being in the place that brought all of us so much happiness together.

While we were there, the owners of the home where we stayed planted several rose bushes (my mom's favorite flower) in my mom's honor. We explained to all of the six grandchildren what we were going to do, and our entire family gathered around the planting area and celebrated my mom's legacy together as each rose bush was placed in the ground. As I said earlier, ALS may take a life but does not necessarily end a relationship. I hope that your relationships live on, too.

References

Below is a list of organizations and references that I found helpful during this journey.

⌣⁀

- Organizations
  - The ALS Association / www.alsa.org
  - The Muscular Dystrophy Association / www.mda.org
  - SeniorBridge Home Care / www.seniorbridge.com
- Reference Materials
  - Mitsumoto, Hiroshi, MD. 2009. *Amyotrophic Lateral Sclerosis: A Guide for Patients and Families*, Third edition. New York: Demos Medical Publishing.
- Other Materials
  - Albom, Mitch. 1997. *Tuesdays with Morrie*. New York: Doubleday.

---

i   The ALS Association, *Facts You Should Know*, http:// www.alsa.org
ii   http:// www.alsa.org
iii Mitch Albom, *Tuesdays with Morrie*, (New York: Doubleday, 1997), 202

www.ingramcontent.com/pod-product-compliance
Lightning Source LLC
Chambersburg PA
CBHW070816290526
45795CB00002B/731